TIGER WOODS:

the making of a legend

Cynthia D. Mora

Copyright page

Table of content

INTRODUCTION

Few names in golf evoke more reverence and awe than Tiger Woods. From the tender age when he first gripped a club until the grand stages of championship victories, Few names in golf evoke more reverence and awe than Tiger Woods. Tiger Woods' journey is not only one of sporting excellence, but also of determination, resilience, and unparalleled talent.

Tiger Woods was born on December 30, 1975, in Cypress, California, with his destiny seemingly predetermined. Tiger was introduced to golf by his father

Earl, himself a passionate golfer, and he demonstrated an innate gift for the game that would soon captivate the world. yet, behind the poised swings and strategic brilliance lay a story of discipline and dedication rarely witnessed in the sporting world

As we delve into Tiger Woods' life, we discover the complexities of his meteoric rise, from his amateur days dominating junior tournaments to his historic victories on the professional tour. Beyond the fairways and greens, Tiger's journey is characterized by personal trials and tribulations, demonstrating the human spirit's ability to endure and overcome.

In this investigation, we hope to uncover the essence of Tiger Woods: the man, the myth, and the legend. From

Tiger Woods

his unrivaled dominance on the golf course to the
tumultuous chapters of his personal life, every aspect of
Tiger's story is a source of inspiration and a reminder of
the heights that can be reached with unwavering focus
and relentless ambition.

Join us as we embark on the oddity through the life and
time of Tiger Woods, a journey that transcends the
boundaries of sports and delves into the heart of
greatness

CHAPTER ONE: WHO IS TIGER WOODS

Tiger Woods is a well-known professional golfer who is regarded as one of the best of all time. Eldrick Tont Woods, born on December 30, 1975, in Cypress, California, rose to prominence early in his career due to his exceptional talent and achievements in the sport. Woods turned professional in 1996 and quickly rose to prominence, winning multiple major championships and breaking numerous records along the way. Throughout his career, he has amassed an impressive collection of awards, including 15 major championships, second only to Jack Nicklaus. Woods' influence extends beyond the golf course, as he has helped popularize the sport and inspired countless people around the world. Despite facing personal and professional challenges, his perseverance and dedication to the game have solidified his status as a sporting icon

1.1 early life

Tiger Woods was born on December 30, 1975, in Cypress, California, to Earl Woods, a retired lieutenant colonel in the United States Army, and Kultida Woods, who is of Thai, Chinese, and Dutch heritage. Tiger demonstrated exceptional talent for golf at a young age, displaying remarkable skill and focus on the course. Tiger's father, Earl, recognized his son's potential and began teaching him the fundamentals of golf when he was a toddler. Tiger developed a disciplined practice routine and a competitive spirit under Earl's tutelage, both of which served him well throughout his career.

Tiger's early years were characterized by a mix of natural talent, rigorous training, and familial support. By the age of three, he was already demonstrating his golfing prowess on television talk shows, enthralling audiences with his early abilities. At the age of five, he was featured in Golf Digest, demonstrating his ability to drive the ball long distances.

Despite his growing talent, Tiger's childhood was not without difficulties. He faced racial discrimination on golf courses as a result of his mixed heritage, an experience that shaped his perspective and advocacy efforts. Tiger, on the other hand, persevered, honing his craft and aspiring to be a professional golfer, thanks to his parents' unwavering support and father's guidance.

Tiger's dedication to the sport was clear throughout his early years. He spent countless hours practicing, often under the watchful eye of his father, who taught him the value of mental toughness and strategic thinking. By the time he reached adolescence, Tiger had established himself as a dominant force in junior golf, winning numerous amateur tournaments and attracting the attention of college recruiters and professional scouts alike.

Tiger's early life was defined by his singular focus on golf, which laid the groundwork for the incredible career that followed. His rise from child prodigy to global sports icon is due to his exceptional talent, unwavering determination, and the formative influence of his upbringing.

1.2 background

Tiger Woods comes from a diverse background, shaped by his family's heritage and upbringing in a supportive but demanding environment.

Earl Woods, Tiger's father, was a retired lieutenant colonel in the United States Army who was known for his disciplined approach to life and served as his primary golf instructor and mentor. Earl instilled in Tiger a strong work ethic, resilience, and strategic mindset that would serve him well both on and off the golf course.

Kultida Woods, Tiger's mother, is of Thai, Chinese, and Dutch descent. She had a significant impact on Tiger's upbringing, offering emotional support and encouragement throughout his journey.

Growing up in a multicultural household exposed Tiger to a variety of perspectives and experiences that shaped his worldview. He experienced racial discrimination at a young age, including prejudice on golf courses due to his mixed heritage. These experiences would later motivate him to advocate for diversity and inclusion in golf and beyond.

Tiger's background includes a strong emphasis on education and personal growth. Despite his early success in golf, his parents emphasized the value of education and character development. Tiger attended Stanford University, where he studied economics while also excelling on the golf course.

Tiger Woods' background is marked by a combination of cultural influences, familial support, and an unwavering pursuit of excellence. These factors have contributed significantly to his identity as a golfer, public figure, and philanthropist.

1.3 education

Tiger Woods went to Western High School in Anaheim, California, where he continued to excel academically while honing his golf skills. Despite his growing success in the sport, he remained focused on his studies, striking a balance between athletics and academics.

After graduating from high school in 1994, Woods attended Stanford University on a golf scholarship. He studied economics while competing for Stanford's golf team, the Cardinals. Despite the demands of his collegiate golf career, Woods prioritized his education, striving for success both on and off the course.

Woods won numerous collegiate golf titles while at Stanford, including the NCAA individual golf championship in 1996. His success at the collegiate level cemented his status as a rising star in the sport.

In 1996, Woods decided to turn professional and forego his remaining two years of eligibility at Stanford. While he did not complete his degree at Stanford, his time there provided him with a solid foundation in academics and personal development, which influenced his multifaceted approach to life and golf.

Throughout his career, Woods has emphasized the value of education and personal development. He has supported a variety of educational initiatives and scholarship programs, recognizing the transformative power of education and the opportunities it offers future generations.

Chapter two: Introduction to golf

Tiger Woods' introduction to golf began at a very young age, influenced by his father, Earl Woods, who recognized his son's natural talent and potential for the game. Earl, a retired lieutenant colonel in the United States Army, introduced Tiger to golf when he was a toddler, giving him a miniature golf club and encouraging him to swing.

Tiger displayed an uncanny ability to play golf from the start, demonstrating an impressive combination of hand-eye coordination, focus, and determination. Under Earl's guidance, Tiger began diligently practicing, honing his skills on the family's backyard golf course and participating in junior tournaments at local clubs.

As Tiger's talent became more apparent, Earl took a disciplined and strategic approach to his son's development, teaching him the fundamentals of the game while emphasizing the value of mental toughness and perseverance. Tiger's early golf experiences laid the groundwork for his future success, influencing his understanding of the game and approach to competition.

Despite facing challenges such as racial discrimination and skepticism from some members of the golfing community, Tiger remained committed to his pursuit of excellence. His passion for golf grew stronger as he grew older, fueling his desire to compete at the highest levels of the sport.

By the time Tiger reached adolescence, he had established himself as a dominant force in junior golf, winning numerous titles and attracting the attention of both college recruiters and professional scouts. His introduction to golf had grown into a full-fledged passion, laying the groundwork for the extraordinary career that followed.

2.1 early interest

Tiger Woods

Tiger Woods' early interest in golf was sparked by his father, Earl Woods, who introduced him to the game at a very young age. Recognizing his son's innate talent and potential, Earl gave Tiger his first set of clubs and began teaching him the fundamentals of the game.

Tiger displayed a natural affinity for golf from the moment he first picked up a club, with remarkable hand-eye coordination and an insatiable desire to improve. He practiced his swing for hours in the family garage and backyard, eagerly absorbing his father's lessons.

Tiger's interest in golf grew, and so did his determination to master the game. He embraced the game's challenges with enthusiasm, constantly looking for ways to improve his technique and performance. Tiger developed a disciplined practice routine and a competitive spirit under Earl's tutelage, both of which served him well throughout his career.

Tiger's early interest in golf was more than just a hobby; it was a passion that consumed him completely. His relentless pursuit of excellence and unwavering dedication to the sport distinguished him from his peers, laying the groundwork for the extraordinary success that would define his professional career.

2.2 training

Tiger Woods

Tiger Woods' training regimen began at a young age and was marked by discipline, dedication, and an unwavering pursuit of perfection. Tiger Woods began a structured and intensive training program under the supervision of his father, Earl Woods, to improve his golf skills and mental fortitude.

Tiger began honing his golf skills at the age of two, spending hours every day practicing his swing and learning the intricacies of the game. Earl, a skilled golfer and retired lieutenant colonel in the United States Army, instilled in his son a strong work ethic and a drive for excellence.

Tiger's training included a wide range of activities, such as technical instruction, physical conditioning, and mental preparation. He worked tirelessly to perfect his technique, meticulously analyzing every detail of his swing and looking for ways to improve his performance.

In addition to his on-course training, Tiger did a variety of off-course exercises to improve his physical strength, flexibility, and endurance. He added weightlifting, cardiovascular workouts, and flexibility drills to his routine, understanding the importance of staying in peak physical condition for competitive success.

Equally important was Tiger's mental preparation, which included visualization techniques, goal setting, and mental conditioning exercises. He developed a mindset of unwavering focus, resilience, and self-belief, preparing him to face the challenges and pressures of professional competition with confidence and poise.

Tiger's dedication to training was unwavering throughout his career, propelling him to unprecedented levels of success in golf. His unwavering commitment to his craft and relentless pursuit of excellence demonstrate the transformative power of disciplined training and unwavering determination.

2.3 Amateur Career Highlights

Tiger Woods

Tiger Woods' amateur career was full of highlights and accomplishments that demonstrated his exceptional talent and laid the groundwork for his future success in professional golf. Here are a few notable highlights from Tiger's amateur career:

1. Junior Golf Dominance: Tiger dominated the junior golf scene from a young age, winning numerous tournaments and championships throughout his childhood. His dominance in junior golf tournaments predicted his future success as a professional golfer. Tiger Woods' dominance in junior golf was nothing short of remarkable, foreshadowing his future success on the professional tour. Tiger Woods demonstrated prodigious talent and an insatiable desire for victory from a young age, capturing the attention of the golfing world with his precocious skills and competitive spirit.

Tiger Woods

Tiger amassed an impressive collection of titles and accolades during his junior golf career, cementing his status as one of the sport's most dominant young talents. His ability to consistently outperform his peers and excel under pressure distinguished him from the competition and predicted his future as a golf prodigy.

Among his notable achievements in junior golf are:

i. Multiple Junior World Championships: Tiger won several titles at the prestigious Junior World Golf Championships, demonstrating his ability to compete and win on a global scale. His victories in this highly competitive event cemented his status as a rising golf star.

ii. U.S. Junior Amateur Success: Tiger's most notable junior golf victory came at the U.S. Junior Amateur Championship, where he won three times in a row from 1991 to 1993, making history. His dominance in this prestigious event demonstrated his exceptional talent and competitive spirit.

iii. AJGA Player of the Year: Tiger was named the American Junior Golf Association (AJGA) Player of the Year several times during his junior golf career, recognizing his consistent performance and impact on the junior golf circuit. His ability to excel in elite junior tournaments cemented his reputation as a future star in the sport.

iv. National and Regional Titles: In addition to his success in major junior golf championships, Tiger won numerous national and regional titles during his junior career. His ability to win across multiple competitions demonstrated his versatility and skill as a golfer.

Tiger's dominance in junior golf earned him widespread recognition and admiration, as well as laying the groundwork for his future success as a professional golfer. During his formative years, his unparalleled talent, work ethic, and competitive drive propelled him to become one of the greatest athletes in the sport's history.

2. Three Consecutive U.S. Junior Amateur Titles: Tiger made history by winning the U.S. Junior Amateur

Championship three years in a row, from 1991 to 1993. This unprecedented feat cemented his reputation as one of the sport's most promising young players.

Tiger Woods' unprecedented success in junior golf culminated in a historic accomplishment: winning three consecutive U.S. Junior Amateur titles from 1991 to 1993. This remarkable achievement cemented his status as one of the sport's most dominant young talents, demonstrating his exceptional skill, determination, and competitive drive.

Winning a single U.S. Junior Amateur title is an impressive accomplishment in and of itself, but Tiger's ability to win the championship three times in a row distinguished him from his peers and earned him widespread acclaim in the golfing community.

Tiger Woods

During his reign as U.S. Junior Amateur champion, Tiger demonstrated exceptional talent and mental fortitude, consistently outperforming his opponents and displaying maturity and composure beyond his years. His victory in this prestigious event foreshadowed his future success on the professional circuit, cementing his reputation as a golfing prodigy.

Tiger's three consecutive U.S. Junior Amateur championships remain a watershed moment in his illustrious career, demonstrating his unrivaled ability to rise to the occasion and achieve greatness on the golf course.

3. Three Consecutive U.S. Amateur Titles: Following his success in junior golf, Tiger extended his winning streak to the collegiate level, winning three consecutive U.S. Amateur Championships from 1994 to 1996. These victories demonstrated his ability to compete against top-tier competition and solidified his status as a future professional golf star.

4. Stanford University Career: While attending Stanford University on a golf scholarship, Tiger further distinguished himself by excelling on the collegiate golf team. In 1994, he led Stanford to victory in the NCAA team championship while also winning the individual NCAA championship. Tiger Woods' college career at Stanford University was nothing short of remarkable, both academically and athletically. Despite his already burgeoning golf career, Woods chose to pursue a college education.

Tiger Woods

Tiger left an indelible mark at Stanford, both academically and athletically. On the golf course, he led the Stanford Cardinal to victory in the 1994 NCAA team championship, demonstrating his leadership abilities and competitive spirit. Individually, he won the NCAA championship the same year, cementing his reputation as one of the country's best amateur golfers.

Off the course, Tiger continued to excel academically, pursuing an economics degree while juggling the demands of collegiate golf. Despite the difficulties of balancing athletics and academics, he demonstrated an exceptional ability to manage his time and maintain high levels of performance in both areas.

Tiger's collegiate career at Stanford gave him invaluable experiences and opportunities for personal and professional development. His time at university allowed him to form lifelong friendships, learn important life skills, and improve his golfing abilities in a competitive and supportive environment.

Tiger Woods' time at Stanford University was marked by success both on and off the golf course. His collegiate achievements laid the groundwork for his future success as a professional golfer, demonstrating his dedication to academic achievement and athletic excellence.

5. Low Amateur at the Masters: In 1995, Tiger Woods made his Masters Tournament debut as an amateur and made an immediate impact by finishing as the low amateur. His impressive performance at Augusta National Golf Club predicted his future success at the

highest levels of professional golf. Tiger Woods made his Masters Tournament debut as an amateur in 1995, and despite being his first time at Augusta National Golf Club, he made an impression. Woods finished the tournament as the lowest amateur, a remarkable achievement for any young golfer, especially on such a prestigious stage.

His performance at the Masters Tournament demonstrated his exceptional talent and ability to compete at the highest levels of professional golf, despite being an amateur. Woods' skill and poise under pressure earned him widespread praise and marked the start of what would become a legendary career in the sport.

While he did not win the tournament as a low amateur, Woods' performance at the Masters demonstrated his potential and foreshadowed the numerous victories and records he would go on to achieve in the years that followed. His performance at Augusta National cemented his status as one of golf's most promising young talents, laying the groundwork for his future PGA Tour dominance.

6. Rising Amateur Ranking: Throughout his amateur career, Tiger held the top spot in the World Amateur Golf Ranking, cementing his position as the world's best amateur golfer. His consistent success on the amateur circuit fueled widespread speculation about his eventual transition to the professional ranks. Tiger Woods' rise in the amateur golf rankings was meteoric, thanks to his exceptional on-course performance and dominance in prestigious tournaments. As he continued to win and

receive accolades, his standing in the amateur golf world grew, cementing his reputation as one of the game's top talents.

Throughout his junior and amateur careers, Tiger's outstanding performances in high-profile events such as the US Junior Amateur Championship and the US Amateur Championship propelled him to the top of the rankings. His ability to consistently outperform his competitors and deliver under pressure gained him widespread recognition and acclaim in the golfing community.

With each victory, Tiger's World Amateur Golf Ranking (WAGR) rose steadily, reflecting his unwavering dedication to excellence and relentless pursuit of success. His rise in the amateur rankings foreshadowed his future dominance on the professional circuit, pointing to an extraordinary career ahead.

Tiger Woods' amateur career was characterized by unprecedented success, numerous championships, and a level of dominance uncommon in the world of golf. His accomplishments during this formative period paved the way for his historic professional career and cemented his legacy as one of golf's greatest players of all time.

CHAPTER THREE: PROFESSIONAL CAREER BEGINNINGS

Tiger Woods' professional career began with much fanfare in August 1996, when he made his PGA Tour debut at the Greater Milwaukee Open. Woods was only 20 years old at the time, having recently decided to forego his final two years of college eligibility at Stanford University to pursue a professional career.

Despite the high expectations surrounding his debut, Woods struggled to find his footing and missed the cut in his first professional tournament. However, he quickly recovered and demonstrated his potential in subsequent events, including a tie for fifth at the 1996 Las Vegas Invitational.

Woods' breakthrough came in April 1997 at the Masters Tournament, when he became the youngest player ever to win the prestigious major championship at the age of 21. His dominant performance at Augusta National Golf Club wowed the world and cemented his place as golf's newest superstar.

Following his historic Masters victory, Woods continued to make waves on the PGA Tour, winning multiple tournaments and receiving widespread praise for his exceptional talent and competitive prowess. His professional debut signaled the start of a new era in golf, as he quickly rose to become one of the sport's most dominant and influential players.

Tiger Woods' professional career started with a combination of prodigious talent, unwavering determination, and unprecedented success. His early PGA Tour achievements paved the way for a legendary career that would reshape the golf landscape and inspire future generations of players.

3.1 turning pro

Tiger Woods' decision to turn professional was a watershed moment in his career and the sport of golf. After an illustrious amateur career that included three consecutive U.S. Amateur titles, Woods announced his decision to forego his remaining two years of Stanford University eligibility to pursue a professional golf career.

Tiger Woods officially turned professional on August 29, 1996, when he signed endorsement deals with Nike and Titleist worth record-breaking sums at the time. His decision to enter the professional ranks was met with great anticipation and excitement, with golf fans and industry insiders looking forward to the young prodigy's PGA Tour debut.

Tiger Woods

Woods made an immediate impact on the professional circuit, playing in his first PGA Tour event, the Greater Milwaukee Open, just days after turning pro. Despite initially struggling to find his rhythm and missing the cut in his debut tournament, Woods quickly adjusted to the pressures of professional golf and began to demonstrate his immense talent and potential.

In October 1996, just months after turning pro, Woods won his first PGA Tour event at the Las Vegas Invitational, ushering in what would become a historic career. His meteoric rise to the top of the golfing world captivated spectators and propelled the sport to new heights of popularity and excitement.

Tiger Woods' decision to turn professional marked the start of a legendary journey that would see him rewrite the record books, dominate the world of golf, and become one of sports' most iconic figures of all time. His impact on the sport and future generations of golfers is still felt today.

3.2: Major wins

Tiger Woods

1. Masters Tournament (Augusta National Golf Club):

  - 1997, 2001, 2002, 2005

2. U.S. Open (various venues):

  - 2000, 2002, 2008

3. The Open Championship (various venues):

  - 2000, 2005, 2006

4. PGA Championship (various venues):

Tiger Woods

- 1999, 2000, 2006, 2007

Woods' major championship wins spanned a decade and included victories on some of the world's most iconic and challenging courses. His ability to perform under pressure and elevate his game on the biggest stages distinguished him from his competitors, earning him admiration and respect from both fans and fellow golfers.

Each major victory strengthened Woods' legacy and cemented his place in golf history. His unparalleled success in major championships remains a defining feature of his remarkable career, inspiring awe and admiration among golf fans all over the world.

3.3 breakthroughs

Tiger Woods' breakthrough moment in professional golf occurred at the 1997 Masters Tournament at Augusta National Golf Club. At the age of 21, Woods made history as the youngest player to win the prestigious major championship, a victory that would forever change the landscape of golf.

Woods, who came into the tournament with a lot of hype and expectations, outperformed them all with his dominant performance. He demonstrated his prodigious talent and unwavering confidence throughout the event, captivating audiences with his exceptional skill and strategic brilliance on the course.

Throughout the tournament, Woods demonstrated a level of dominance rarely seen in the sport, consistently outperforming his opponents and pulling away from the pack. His remarkable combination of power, precision, and composure under pressure propelled him to a record-breaking victory with a commanding 12-stroke lead, the largest in Masters history.

Woods' breakthrough victory at the 1997 Masters Tournament was more than just a golfing triumph; it was a cultural phenomenon that went beyond the sport. His historic victory broke down racial barriers and inspired a new generation of athletes from various backgrounds to pursue their goals in golf and beyond.

The significance of Woods' breakthrough victory at the Masters cannot be overemphasized. It signaled the start of a new era in golf, as he emerged as a transcendent figure capable of transcending the game and captivating the world with his talent, charisma, and undeniable impact.

3.4 Dominance.

Tiger Woods

Tiger Woods' dominance in the world of golf is unparalleled and has lasted over two decades. From the late 1990s to the mid-2000s, Woods redefined the game with his unrivaled skill, mental toughness, and relentless pursuit of perfection. His dominance can be seen in a variety of aspects of the game:

1. Major Championships: Woods' record at major championships speaks for itself. He has won 15 major titles, second only to Jack Nicklaus. Woods' ability to perform at the highest level on golf's most prestigious stages, such as the Masters, U.S. Open, The Open Championship, and PGA Championship, cemented his legacy as one of the greatest major champions in history.

2. PGA Tour Wins: Woods' dominance on the PGA Tour is unparalleled. He has won an incredible 82 PGA Tour events, tying Sam Snead for the most all-time. Woods' consistency and ability to win tournaments on a variety of courses, conditions, and formats demonstrate his dominance in professional golf.

3. World Number One Ranking: Woods spent a record 683 weeks as the world's number one golfer. His ability to remain at the top of the rankings for such an extended period demonstrates his dominance over his peers as well as his long-term success.

4. Winning Streaks: Throughout his career, Woods had several notable winning streaks, including his well-known "Tiger Slam" in 2000-2001, during which he

held all four major titles concurrently. He also had streaks of consecutive cuts and weeks ranked as world number one, demonstrating his dominance in the sport.

5. Impact on the Game: In addition to his achievements, Woods has had a significant impact on the game of golf. He popularized the sport on a global scale, bringing in new fans and participants from various backgrounds. His influence extends to television ratings, prize money, and sponsorship deals, propelling the sport to unprecedented heights of popularity and visibility.

Tiger Woods' dominance in golf is more than just winning tournaments; it's about how he transformed the sport, raised the bar for competition, and inspired generations of players to strive for greatness. His legacy as a dominant force in golf will be felt for generations to come.

3.5 records

Tiger Woods has set numerous golf records, many of which are regarded as benchmarks of excellence and dominance in the sport. Here are some of his most notable recordings:

1. Major Championship Wins: Tiger Woods has won fifteen major championships, including:

- Five Masters Tournament victories.

Tiger Woods

- Three United States Open titles

- Three Open Championships

- Four PGA Championships

2. Consecutive Cuts: Woods has made the most consecutive cuts on the PGA Tour, 142 from 1998 to 2005.

3. World Number One Ranking: Woods was ranked as the world's number one golfer for 683 weeks, the most by any player in history.

4. Most Consecutive Weeks Ranked World Number One: Woods also has the record for the most consecutive weeks ranked as the world's number one golfer, 281 from June 12, 2005, to October 30, 2010.

5. Youngest Golfer to Achieve Career Grand Slam: At the age of 24, Woods became the youngest golfer to complete the career Grand Slam (winning all four major championships).

6. Lowest Scoring Average in a Season: In 2000, Woods had the lowest scoring average on the PGA Tour, averaging 68.17 strokes per round.

7. Largest Margin of Victory in Masters Tournament History: Tiger Woods' 12-stroke victory at the 1997 Masters Tournament is the tournament's largest margin of victory.

These records, among others, demonstrate Tiger Woods' extraordinary talent, dominance, and influence on the game of golf. His achievements cemented his legacy as one of the greatest athletes of all time, leaving an indelible mark on the game's history.

Chapter four: peak years

Tiger Woods' stylish times in golf are extensively regarded as being from the late 1990s to the mid-2000s. During this time, Woods achieved unknown success, cementing his position as one of the sport's most dominant athletes. Some of the main highlights and accomplishments from his peak times are

1. Major Major Championship Wins During this time, Woods won the maturity of his 15 major crowns, including his well- known" Tiger Slam" in 2000- 2001, in which he held all four major titles. Tiger Woods'

major major crown palms demonstrate his unequaled skill, internal fiber, and dominance in the world of golf. Woods has won 15 major crowns in his outstanding career, cementing his heritage as one of the topmost golfers of all time. This are some of his memorable 1997 Masters events

i. At the age of 21, Woods became the youngest player in history to win the Masters. His dominant performance at Augusta National Golf Club, which included a record-breaking 12- stroke palm, charmed golf suckers around the world.

ii. 2000U.S. Open Woods demonstrated his complete dominance at the 2000U.S. Open, which was held at Pebble Beach Golf Links. He delivered a masterful performance, winning the event by a stunning 15 strokes, the largest margin of the palm in US Open history.

iii. 2000 Open Championship Woods continued his remarkable run of success in 2000, winning the Open

Championship at St Andrews' Old Course. His palm completed the career Grand Slam, making him the youthful player to do so at the age of 24.

iv. 2000 PGA Championship In a major season, Woods won his third major title, the PGA Championship, at Valhalla Golf Club. His palm limited off an inconceivable run of success, earning him the surname" Tiger Slam" for contemporaneously holding all four major titles. In the 2005 Masters Tournament Woods won his fourth green jacket with a memorable playoff palm over Chris DiMarco. His palm marked a triumphant return to form after a lengthy failure in major crowns, cementing his place as one of the game's greats.

vi. 2008 US Open Despite suffering a knee injury that needed surgery, Woods won the 2008 US Open at Torrey Pines, demonstrating his fabulous adaptability. His dramatic playoff palm over Rocco Mediate, despite violent pain, demonstrated his unvarying determination and internal fiber. These major major crown palms give only a regard into Tiger Woods' remarkable career and lasting heritage in the world of golf. His capability to rise to the occasion on golf's biggest stages and deliver clutch performances under pressure has left an unforgettable mark on the game and continues to inspire unborn generations of players.

2. World Number One Dominance Woods spent a record- breaking 683 weeks as the world's number one golfer, the maturity of which passed during his peak times. Tiger Woods' dominance as the world's top golfer is unknown in the sport's history. Woods has been ranked as the world's number one golfer for an aggregate of 683 weeks, a record that demonstrates his harmonious excellence and unequaled success in the PGA stint.   Woods' capability to remain the world's stylish golfer for so long is a testament to his remarkable thickness, skill, and internal durability. Throughout his time as the top- ranked player, Woods continued to win, set records, and dominate the competition, cementing his place as one of the topmost athletes of all time.   His reign as world number one gauged several ages of golf,

as he faced competition from a new generation of talented players. Nevertheless, Woods remained the standard of excellence, setting the bar for success and inspiring admiration and admiration from both suckers and challengers. Woods' reign as the world's top golfer not only cemented his heritage as one of the sport's topmost players but also raised golf's global profile. His influence on the game extended beyond individual accomplishments, as he brought unknown attention and excitement to golf, attracting new suckers and propelling the sport to new heights. Overall, Tiger Woods' dominance as the world's stylish golfer is a dcfining point of his fabulous career, demonstrating his unequaled gift, fidelity, and impact on the sport of golf.

3. an unexampled PGA Tour Success Woods has won multitudinous PGA Tour events, including several Player of the Year awards and FedEx Cup crowns. He also had several winning stripes and established records for successive cuts and the lowest- scoring normal in a season. Tiger Woods' PGA Tour success is unequaled , and his name will go down in golf history for his

extraordinary achievements. Throughout his outstanding career, Woods won an inconceivable 82 PGA Tour events, tying Sam Snead for the most wins in PGA Tour history. Several factors contribute to his unequaled success on the PGA Tour, including:

i.his capability to constantly perform at a high position distinguished him from his challengers. Whether he was winning major crowns or dominating regular stint events, Woods was remarkably harmonious throughout his career.

ii. Versatility Woods demonstrated his versatility by winning events under a variety of formats, courses, and conditions. From traditional stroke- play events to match- play competitions, Woods demonstrated his capability to excel in any situation and acclimatize his game to changing challenges.

iii. Mental Toughness: Woods' mental toughness and ability to thrive under pressure contributed significantly to his PGA Tour success. He had a steely resolve and unwavering confidence, allowing him to deliver clutch performances in critical moments.

iv. Record-Breaking Streaks: Throughout his PGA Tour career, Woods had several record-breaking streaks, including his incredible run of 142 consecutive cuts from 1998-2005. He also established records for consecutive weeks as the world's number-one golfer and lowest-scoring average in a season.

v. Impact on the Sport: Woods' success on the PGA Tour transformed the sport of golf by attracting new fans, increasing television ratings, and raising the level of competition. His captivating playing style and magnetic personality elevated him to the status of a global icon and contributed to the global popularity of golf.

Overall, Tiger Woods' unparalleled success on the PGA Tour is a testament to his exceptional talent, work ethic, and determination. His legacy as one of the greatest golfers of all time is firmly established and his impact on the field will be felt for generations to come

4. Cultural Impact: Woods' success went beyond golf, making him a global icon. He became one of the world's most recognizable and marketable athletes, with endorsements, sponsorships, and widespread media coverage raising the sport's profile.

Tiger Woods' cultural impact extends beyond golf to include other sports, entertainment, and society as a whole. His impact has been profound and far-reaching, with an indelible mark on many aspects of modern culture. Here are some important ways Tiger Woods has made a cultural impact:

Tiger Woods

In i. Diversity and Representation: As one of his generation's most successful and recognizable athletes, Woods broke down racial barriers and challenged stereotypes in golf, a predominantly white sport. His success as a person of mixed-racial heritage inspired people from various backgrounds to pursue careers in golf and other sports, paving the way for increased diversity and representation in athletics.

ii. Globalization of Golf: Woods' international appeal and popularity contributed to golf's global popularity. His success cut across borders and cultures, bringing new fans and participants to the sport from all over the world. As a result, golf experienced a surge in popularity in regions where it was previously less visible, contributing to its status as a truly global phenomenon

iii. Mainstream Media Attention: Woods' celebrity status and magnetic personality made him a regular in mainstream media outlets, reaching audiences outside of the traditional golfing demographic. His appearances in television commercials, magazine covers, and talk shows boosted golf's profile and introduced the sport to previously uninterested audiences.

iv. Economic Impact: Woods' influence extended beyond the golf course into the world of business and commerce. His endorsement deals with major brands like Nike, Gatorade, and Rolex resulted in significant revenue and increased sales of golf equipment, apparel, and accessories. Furthermore, his participation in tournaments and events helped to boost tourism and economic activity in the host cities.

v. Philanthropy and Social Causes: Woods' philanthropic efforts and participation in charitable initiatives have positively impacted society. His Tiger Woods Foundation has funded educational programs, youth development initiatives, and community outreach efforts aimed at empowering underprivileged youth and promoting social change.

Overall, Tiger Woods' cultural impact is multifaceted and long-lasting, reflecting his status as a global icon and symbol of excellence, perseverance, and success. His legacy extends beyond sports, leaving an indelible mark on contemporary culture.

5. Revolutionizing the Game: Woods' dominance and style of play transformed the sport of golf. He elevated the sport's athleticism, power, and mental toughness, inspiring a generation of young golfers and reshaping the way it is played and perceived. Tiger Woods transformed golf from a niche sport to a mainstream cultural phenomenon. His impact on the game can be seen in a variety of ways, including:

i. Athleticism and Fitness: Woods brought a new level of athleticism to golf, challenging the stereotype of golfers as unathletic individuals. His strict fitness regimen and emphasis on strength and conditioning influenced a new generation of golfers to prioritize physical fitness and athleticism in their training regimens.

ii. Power and Distance: Woods changed the way golf was played by demonstrating his incredible power and driving distance off the tee. His ability to hit the ball for long distances with precision and control compelled course designers to reconsider course layouts and adapt to the modern game.

iii. Mental Toughness: Woods' mental toughness and competitive mindset established a new standard for golf success. His unwavering focus, resilience in the face of adversity, and ability to perform under pressure pushed the boundaries of what it means to be a successful golfer.

iv. Globalization and Diversity: Woods' diverse background and international appeal contributed to the globalization of golf, bringing in new fans and participants from all over the world. His success encouraged people from all walks of life to play golf and challenged stereotypes about who could excel at it.

v. Media and Sponsorship: Woods' charisma, marketability, and star power catapulted golf into a popular spectator sport and lucrative business venture. His media appearances, endorsement deals with major brands, and high-profile tournaments all contributed to golf's rise in popularity and appeal to new audiences.

vi. Youth Participation: Woods' early success and relatability to younger audiences contributed to an increase in youth golf participation. His foundation's initiatives to promote youth development and access to the sport have motivated countless young golfers to pursue their goals.

Overall, Tiger Woods has had a profound and far-reaching impact on the game of golf, shaping it in ways that can still be felt today. His legacy as a trailblazer, innovator, and ambassador for the game will last for generation

Chapter Five: Major Championship

Major championships in golf are widely regarded as the pinnacle of the sport, attracting the best players from all over the world to compete for prestigious titles on legendary courses. Professional golf features four major championships:

1. The Masters Tournament: The Masters, held annually at Augusta National Golf Club in Augusta, Georgia, is the year's first major championship and, arguably, the most prestigious. It is famous for its tradition, history, and the iconic green jacket presented to the champion. The Masters Tournament, commonly known as "The

Masters," is one of the most prestigious events in professional golf. It is held annually at the Augusta National Golf Club in Augusta, Georgia, usually during the first full week of April.

The Masters is renowned for its rich history, storied traditions, and storied champions, making it a highlight of the golfing calendar and a must-watch event for golf enthusiasts around the world.

2. U.S. Open: The U.S. Open, organized by the United States Golf Association (USGA), is distinguished by its demanding course layouts and difficult conditions. It is traditionally held on various courses across the United States and has a reputation for determining the best overall golfer. The US Open is one of professional golf's four major championships, organized by the United States Golf Association (USGA). The following are some key features and characteristics of the US Open:

i. Course Selection: The U.S. Open is held on a rotating basis at prestigious golf courses across the country. The USGA carefully selects these courses because of their challenging layouts and ability to put the world's best golfers to the test. Some iconic US Open venues include Pebble Beach.

ii. Championship Format: The U.S. Open is a four-round stroke play tournament with 72 holes spread across four days. The field includes both professional and amateur golfers who have qualified or received exemptions to participate in the event. The player with the lowest total score at the end of the tournament is crowned the U.S. Open winner.

iii. Stringent Course Setup: The USGA is well-known for its stringent course setup at the US Open, which frequently features narrow fairways, thick rough, and lightning-fast greens. The goal is to provide a challenging golf test that requires players to use precision, shot-making ability, and strategic decision-making. Course conditions can be notoriously difficult, and par is an excellent score on many holes.

iv. Signature Trophy: The winner of the US Open is awarded the iconic US Open Championship Trophy, also known as the "U.S. Open Cup" or simply the "Trophy." This prestigious trophy is presented to the champion immediately following the conclusion of the tournament as a symbol of their success in overcoming one of golf's most difficult challenges.

v. Historic Legacy: With a history dating back to 1895, the US Open is one of golf's oldest and most prestigious tournaments. The U.S. Open has produced memorable moments, dramatic finishes, and legendary champions who have left an indelible imprint on the sport.

Overall, the United States Open is a pinnacle event in professional golf, known for its demanding courses grueling competition, and storied legacy that continues to captivate fans around the world

3. Open Championship (British Open) The Open Championship, the oldest of the four major championships, is held each year in the United Kingdom on links-style courses. It is renowned for its unpredictable weather and the strategic challenges posed by natural elements such as wind and undulating terrain.

The Open Championship, also known as the "British Open," is one of professional golf's four major championships, along with the Masters, the United States Open, and the PGA Championship. The following are some key features and characteristics of the Open Championship.

i. Historical Legacy: The Open Championship, the oldest of the four major championships, has a rich history dating back to 1860. It is steeped in tradition, having been played on some of the most historic and iconic links courses in the United Kingdom.

ii. Links-Style Golf: Unlike the other majors, which are usually played on parkland or inland courses, the Open Championship is only played on links courses. Links golf is distinguished by its seaside setting, undulating terrain, and natural hazards such as pot bunkers and unpredictable weather.

iii. Rotating Venues: The Open Championship is played at a variety of prestigious links courses across the United Kingdom. These venues include famous courses like St Andrews, Royal Birkdale, Royal Troon, and Royal St George's. Each course presents distinct challenges and necessitates a different style of play from the competitors.

iv. Claret Jug Trophy: The winner of The Open Championship is awarded the coveted Claret Jug trophy, which is one of golf's most recognizable trophies. The Claret Jug has been awarded to the champion since the tournament's inception, and it represents their triumph over the challenges of links golf.

v. International Field: The Open Championship draws a diverse and international field of competitors, including the world's best professional and amateur golfers. Players from all over the world compete for the chance to play in golf's oldest major championship and be remembered alongside the game's greatest champions.

vi. Dramatic Finishes: The Open Championship has produced some of golf's most memorable and dramatic finishes. From historic duels to miraculous shots, the tournament is known for producing thrilling moments that captivate fans and define the legacies of its winners.

Overall, the Open Championship has a special place in the hearts of golf fans and players alike, revered for its rich history, unique challenges, and unforgettable moments that have elevated it to one of the sport's most prestigious events.

4. PGA Championship: The Professional Golfers' Association of America (PGA) organizes the PGA Championship, which is held at various courses across the United States. It is known for its strong field and competitive format, with winners receiving the prestigious Wanamaker Trophy. The PGA Championship, also known as the "PGA Championship" or simply "the PGA," is one of the four major championships in professional golf. The following are

some key features and characteristics of the PGA Championship:

i. Organized by the PGA of America: Unlike the other three major championships, which are organized by governing bodies (the Masters by Augusta National Golf Club, the US Open by the USGA, and the Open Championship by the R&A), the PGA Championship is organized by the Professional Golfers' Association of America (PGA of America).

ii. Course Selection: The PGA Championship is held at a variety of courses across the United States, each chosen for its ability to provide a difficult test of golf for the world's best players. These courses frequently feature a combination of traditional parkland layouts and more modern designs.

iii. Strong Field: The PGA Championship has traditionally had one of the strongest fields in professional golf, featuring the best players from around the world. The field includes both professional and amateur golfers who have qualified or received exemptions to compete in the events

iv. Major Status: The PGA Championship has been considered one of golf's major championships since 1958. It is regarded as one of the sport's most prestigious events, providing players with the opportunity to compete for a coveted major title and cement their place in golf history.

v. Wanamaker Trophy: The PGA Championship winner is awarded the Wanamaker Trophy, which is named after

Rodman Wanamaker, a key figure in the PGA of America's founding. The Wanamaker Trophy is one of golf's largest and most recognizable trophies, awarded to the winner immediately after the tournament.

vi. Stroke Play Format: The PGA Championship, like the other major championships, is played over four rounds of stroke play, with 72 holes spread across four days. The player with the lowest total score at the end of the tournament is declared the winner.

Overall, the PGA Championship holds a unique place in the world of golf, providing players with the opportunity to compete for a major title and etch their names into golf history. The PGA Championship continues to captivate both fans and players with its strong field, challenging courses, and prestigious traditions.

Winning a major championship is regarded as the pinnacle of professional golf achievement, with players vying to be remembered alongside the game's greatest legends.

Chapter six: off course challenges

Tiger Woods has faced numerous off-course challenges throughout his career, including personal, health, and legal concerns. Some of the major off-course challenges he has faced include:

1. Personal Issues: When reports of marital infidelity surfaced in 2009, Woods' marriage crumbled and he issued a public apology. The scandal harmed his reputation and prompted a period of personal turmoil and introspection.

2. Injuries: Throughout his career, Woods has suffered several injuries, including knee and back problems, which have limited his ability to compete at the highest level. He has undergone multiple surgeries and lengthy rehabilitation processes to address these issues, resulting in extended absences from the game.

3. Legal Issues: Woods has faced legal challenges, including a well-publicized DUI arrest in 2017, which he blamed on the effects of prescription medication. The incident resulted in legal consequences and increased scrutiny of his personal life and pain management issues.

4. Woods' off-course struggles have hurt his public image and reputation, with media attention frequently overshadowing his on-course accomplishments. He has received criticism and speculation from the press and public, as well as scrutiny of his actions and decisions on and off the golf course.

5. Sponsorship and Endorsements: Woods' off-course challenges have had an impact on his sponsorship and endorsement deals, with some companies pulling away from him in the wake of the controversy. While he has lucrative partnerships with brands such as Nike and Rolex, his off-course behavior has occasionally hampered his marketability and appeal to sponsors.

Despite these off-course challenges, Woods has demonstrated courage and determination in overcoming adversity and returning to competitive golf. His ability to handle personal and professional setbacks with grace and perseverance has earned him admiration and respect from both fans and competitors.

6.1 Personal struggles.

Tiger Woods has faced several personal challenges throughout his life and career, including:

1. Marital Issues: When reports of Woods' extramarital affairs surfaced in 2009, he faced intense media scrutiny. This resulted in the public dissolution of his marriage to Elin Nordegren and a period of personal turmoil for Woods.

2. Injuries: Throughout his career, Woods has undergone numerous knee and back surgeries. These injuries have not only limited his ability to compete but have also had an impact on his physical and mental health. Tiger Woods has suffered numerous injuries throughout his illustrious career, which have hampered his performance and kept him out of competition for extended periods. Woods has sustained significant injuries, including:

i. Knee Injuries: Woods has had several knee surgeries, beginning with one to remove fluid and a benign cyst in 1994. He had arthroscopic knee surgery in 2002 to remove fluid and cysts, then reconstructive surgery on his left knee in 2008 to repair a torn ACL and additional cartilage damage.

ii. Back Injuries: Woods has suffered from back problems throughout his career, which began with a herniated disc in 2010. He had microdiscectomy surgery in 2014 and 2015 to relieve pain and pressure on his spine. In 2017, Woods had his fourth back surgery, a spinal fusion, which was successful in relieving his back pain and allowing him to return to competitive golf.

iii. Achilles Tendon: In 2011, Woods injured his left Achilles tendon during the Masters Tournament's third round. While he initially played through the injury, he was eventually forced to withdraw from the tournament and seek medical attention.

iv. Neck Injuries: Woods has experienced neck discomfort and stiffness at various points in his career, which he has attributed to the wear and tear of playing professional golf. While these neck issues have not required surgery, they have contributed to his overall physical discomfort and affected his ability to practice and compete.

iv. Neck Injuries: Woods has experienced neck discomfort and stiffness throughout his career, which he attributes to the wear and tear of professional golf. While these neck issues have not necessitated surgery, they have added to his overall physical discomfort and limited his ability to practice and compete.

These injuries have not only limited Woods' ability to play golf but have also had an impact on his physical health and overall quality of life. Despite these obstacles, Woods has shown remarkable resilience and determination in his efforts to overcome injuries and return to competitive golf at the highest levels.

3. Mental Health: Like many high-profile athletes, Woods has faced mental health challenges, such as the pressure to perform consistently well, dealing with injuries, and dealing with the intense media scrutiny that

comes with being in the spotlight. Tiger Woods has not opened up much about his mental health issues in public. However, like many high-profile athletes, he has most likely faced a variety of pressures and stressors throughout his career, which can have an impact on his mental health. These may include the need to consistently perform at a high level, deal with injuries and setbacks, manage public expectations, and navigate personal and professional relationships while under intense scrutiny.

In addition to the physical toll of injuries and the demands of competition, golf has a significant mental component that requires focus, concentration, and resilience to succeed. Woods has faced numerous challenges on and off the golf course, including personal struggles and setbacks, which have undoubtedly had an impact on his mental health.

While Woods has not spoken extensively about seeking professional help for mental health issues, many athletes and public figures have become more open about their experiences with mental health challenges, reducing stigma and encouraging others to seek help when necessary.

Regardless of the specifics of Woods' mental health journey, his resilience and ability to overcome adversity on and off the golf course are undeniable.

4. Substance Abuse: Since his DUI arrest in 2017, Woods has struggled with prescription medication use and has received addiction treatment. He has been open

about his pain management struggles and the need for help to address them.

5. Family Dynamics: Woods' relationship with his father, Earl Woods, was complicated, and his father's death in 2006 left an indelible mark on him. Woods has also faced the challenges of co-parenting his children with his ex-wife, Elin Nordegren, following their divorce.

Despite his struggles, Woods has demonstrated resilience and perseverance on and off the golf course. He has sought treatment for his problems, worked to rebuild his personal life, and pursued his passion for golf. His ability to overcome adversity while remaining one of the greatest golfers of all time demonstrates his character and determination.

6.2 setbacks.

Tiger Woods has experienced numerous setbacks in his career, both on and off the golf course. Some of the notable setbacks are:

1. Injuries: Throughout his career, Woods has suffered numerous injuries, including knee and back problems, limiting his ability to compete at the highest level. These injuries necessitated surgeries and extensive

rehabilitation, resulting in extended absences from the game and difficulty regaining form upon return.

2. Personal Issues: When reports of marital infidelity surfaced in 2009, Woods' marriage was publicly unraveled, resulting in a period of personal turmoil for him. The scandal harmed his reputation and had an impact on his golf game.

3Woods has had legal issues, including a high-profile DUI arrest in 2017, which he blamed on the effects of prescription medication. The incident resulted in legal consequences and increased scrutiny of his personal life and pain management issues.

4. Performance Decline: Throughout his career, Woods has had periods of poor performance, which were frequently accompanied by injuries and personal issues. He has received criticism and doubts about his ability to compete at the highest level, raising questions about his future in the sport.

Despite these setbacks, Woods demonstrated tenacity and determination in overcoming adversity and returning to competitive golf. He has worked tirelessly to recover from injuries, resolve personal issues, and regain his golfing form.

Chapter seven: comebacks and resurgence

Tiger Woods' comeback and resurgence in golf is one of the most incredible stories in sports history. Despite numerous setbacks, such as injuries, personal challenges, and a drop in performance, Woods has shown incredible resilience and determination in his return to the top of the game. Here are some important aspects of his comeback and resurgence:

Tiger Woods

1. Physical Rehabilitation: After multiple surgeries, including a spinal fusion in 2017, Woods underwent extensive physical therapy to recover from his injuries and regain strength and mobility. He collaborated closely with medical professionals and fitness experts to rebuild his body and prepare for his return to competitive golf. Tiger Woods' physical rehabilitation journey has been an important part of his comeback and resurgence in golf. Here are some key aspects of his rehabilitation

i. Medical Evaluation: Woods collaborated with a team of medical professionals, including orthopedic surgeons, physical therapists, and sports medicine specialists, to determine the severity of his injuries and devise a personalized rehabilitation plan. This included a thorough examination of his musculoskeletal system, range of motion, strength, and functional capabilities.

ii. Post-Surgical Care: After surgery, Woods received specialized post-operative care to help with pain, swelling, and wound healing. Medication, rest, and therapeutic modalities such as ice and heat therapy may have been used to relieve pain and speed up recovery.

iii. Physical Therapy: Woods underwent structured physical therapy sessions to regain mobility, strength, and flexibility in the affected areas of his body, especially his back and lower body. Physical therapists use a variety of techniques, exercises, and manual therapies to correct muscle imbalances, increase joint mobility, and improve overall function.

iv. Progressive Exercise Program: As Woods' rehabilitation progressed, his exercise regimen most likely evolved to include a variety of therapeutic exercises, functional movements, and golf-specific drills. These exercises were intended to gradually increase in intensity and complexity, allowing him to rebuild strength, stability, and proprioception while reducing the risk of re-injury.

v. Core Strengthening: Given the importance of core stability in golf, Woods most likely focused heavily on strengthening his core muscles to support his spine and improve his biomechanics. Core exercises like planks, bridges, and rotational movements may have been included in his rehabilitation program to help him generate power and maintain proper posture during his golf swing.

vi. Cardiovascular Conditioning: In addition to strength training, Woods most likely included cardiovascular exercise in his rehabilitation program to improve his overall fitness and endurance. Walking, cycling, and swimming are all cardiovascular activities that can improve cardiovascular health, promote recovery, and support overall well-being.

vii. Gradual Return to Golf Activities: Throughout his rehabilitation, Woods would have gradually reintroduced golf-specific activities and practice sessions into his schedule. This would have entailed initially focusing on technique, short-game work, and controlled swings before gradually progressing to full-swing practice and tournament competition.

Overall, Tiger Woods' commitment to physical rehabilitation was critical to his ability to overcome injury setbacks and return to top-level competitive golf. His dedication to his recovery, combined with the expertise of his medical team, allowed him to reclaim his physical health and pursue his passion for the game with renewed vigor.

2. Mental Toughness: Woods' mental toughness and competitive spirit were critical factors in his comeback. Despite doubts and setbacks, he remained focused and determined to overcome obstacles and return to form on the golf course. His unwavering confidence in his abilities and dedication to his craft fueled his comeback efforts. Tiger Woods' mental toughness has been a defining characteristic throughout his career, helping him overcome obstacles and achieve success on the golf

course. Here are some important aspects of Woods'
mental toughness:

i. Focus and Concentration: Woods is well-known for his
ability to remain focused and concentrated under
pressure. He has an incredible ability to block out
distractions and remain present in the moment, allowing
him to perform at his peak when it counts the most.

ii. Resilience: Throughout his career, Woods has
overcome numerous setbacks and obstacles, such as
injuries, personal difficulties, and periods of poor
performance. However, he has consistently demonstrated
resilience in the face of adversity, overcoming setbacks
with determination and resolve.

iii. Positive Mindset: Woods approaches challenges with a positive attitude and confidence in his abilities to overcome obstacles. He has a strong sense of self-belief and confidence in his abilities, which allows him to persevere in difficult situations and stay motivated to achieve his goals.

iv. Adaptability: Woods is highly adaptable, adjusting his game plan and strategy in response to changing conditions and circumstances. On the golf course, he excels at problem-solving, coming up with innovative solutions to navigate difficult situations and capitalize on opportunities.

v. Emotional Control: Woods has exceptional emotional control, remaining calm and level-headed even in high-pressure situations. He can effectively manage his emotions, channeling nervous energy and frustration into focused, productive performance.

vi. Competitive Drive: Woods is known for his fierce competitive spirit and desire to win. He thrives on the intensity of competition and welcomes the opportunity to compete against the world's best players. His competitive nature fuels his drive and determination to succeed.

vii. Learning from Failure: Woods sees failure as a chance to grow and learn. He is not afraid to make mistakes or face setbacks, understanding that they are an unavoidable part of the path to excellence. He uses setbacks as motivation to improve and pursue continuous development.

Overall, Tiger Woods' mental toughness is critical to his success as a golfer. His ability to remain focused, resilient, and positive in the face of adversity distinguishes him as one of the best competitors in the sport's history.

3. Strategic Adjustments: As Woods dealt with physical limitations and changes in his game as a result of the injury, he made strategic changes to his golf approach. He worked on improving his overall health and fitness,

fine-tuning his swing mechanics, and adapting his playing style to any physical limitations.

Tiger Woods has made strategic adjustments throughout his career to accommodate changes in his physical condition, competition, and the demands of professional golf. Here are some important strategic adjustments he has made:

i. Swing Changes: Woods has made significant changes to his golf swing over the years, working with various coaches to improve his technique and correct flaws. These modifications have ranged from minor tweaks to major overhauls, aiming to improve consistency, power, and accuracy

ii. Equipment Changes: Woods has regularly experimented with various golf equipment, such as clubs, balls, and shafts, to improve his performance on the course. He has worked closely with equipment manufacturers to tailor his gear to his swing and playing style, leveraging every technological advantage available.

iii. Physical Conditioning: Recognizing the value of fitness in modern golf, Woods has prioritized physical conditioning throughout his career. He has implemented rigorous workout routines to improve strength, flexibility, and endurance, allowing him to generate more power and sustain his performance throughout a round and tournament.

iv. Strategic Course Management: As Woods' game progressed, so did his approach to course management.

He has become more strategic in his shot selection, learning to capitalize on his strengths while minimizing risks and avoiding trouble. This frequently entails taking a more conservative approach off the tee and relying on his precise iron play and short game to score.

v. Schedule Management: In recent years, Woods has changed his tournament schedule to prioritize his health and longevity. He has been more selective about the events he competes in, focusing on peak performance at major championships and key tournaments while strategically managing his workload to avoid overexertion and injury.

vi. Mental Approach: Woods has improved his mental approach to the game, learning how to remain patient, focused, and resilient in the face of adversity. He has developed mental techniques to manage stress, control emotions, and maintain confidence in his abilities, allowing him to perform at his peak when it counts the most.

Overall, Tiger Woods' strategic adjustments have contributed to his continued success and longevity in professional golf. By constantly adapting and evolving his game, he has remained competitive at the highest level while cementing his legacy as one of the greatest players of all time.

4. Success on the Course: Woods' comeback culminated in a historic victory at the 2019 Masters Tournament, where he won his fifth green jacket and 15th major

championship. The victory marked Woods' triumphant return to the winner's circle and cemented his place as one of the greatest golfers of all time. Tiger Woods' golfing success is unprecedented in the sport's history. Throughout his career, he has set numerous milestones and records, cementing his place as one of golf's greatest players of all time. Here are some important highlights of Woods' success on the course:

i. Major Championships: Woods has won a total of 15 major championships, including:

- The Masters: 5 titles (1997, 2001, 2002, 2005, 2019)

- U.S. Open: 3 titles (2000, 2002, 2008)

- The Open Championship (British Open): 3 titles (2000, 2005, 2006)

- PGA Championship: 4 titles (1999, 2000, 2006, 2007)

ii. PGA Tour Wins: Woods has 82 PGA Tour victories, which is the second-highest total in history. His PGA Tour victories include regular tour events, the World Golf Championships (WGC), and the Players Championship.

iii. Career Grand Slam: Woods is one of only five golfers who have won all four major championships at least once in their careers. He completed the Career Grand Slam at the age of 24, making him the youngest player to do so.

iv. Longevity: Woods' golfing success spans two decades, from his professional debut in 1996 to the present. Despite injuries and personal challenges, he has consistently performed at a high level throughout his career.

v. World Number One: Woods has been the world's number one golfer for 683 weeks, the longest streak in PGA Tour history. He has held the number-one spot for more than 13 years, demonstrating his dominance and consistency at the top of the sport.

vi. Unprecedented Dominance: Woods' dominance in the early 2000s is widely regarded as one of the greatest eras in golf history. He won multiple majors in consecutive seasons, held all four major titles at once (the "Tiger

Slam"), and set numerous scoring, margin of victory, and win percentage records.

Tiger Woods' success on the golf course is a reflection of his talent, work ethic, and competitive spirit. His influence on golf has been profound, inspiring generations of players and significantly shaping the modern game.

5. Inspiration and Influence: Woods' comeback has inspired fans and competitors all over the world, demonstrating the importance of perseverance and resilience in the face of adversity. His ability to overcome obstacles and achieve success in the face of setbacks inspires athletes and people from all walks of life. Tiger Woods' influence on the world of golf goes far

beyond his outstanding performance on the course. He has been an inspiration and role model to millions of people around the world, transcending sports and leaving a lasting legacy in a variety of fields. Here are a few ways Woods has inspired and influenced others:

i. Diversity and Inclusion: Woods' success as a biracial golfer has broken down barriers and challenged stereotypes in a predominantly white sport. He has inspired a new generation of diverse golfers to pursue their dreams and has played an important role in promoting diversity and inclusion in the sport.

ii. Global Reach: Woods' worldwide popularity has contributed to the global growth of golf. His electrifying style of play and charismatic personality have drawn fans from all over the world, broadening the sport's reach and appeal to new audiences.

iii. Youth Engagement: Woods' influence on young golfers has been profound, inspiring countless children and teenagers to pick up a club and pursue their interest in the game. His early success has taught aspiring golfers that anything is possible with hard work, dedication, and perseverance.

iv. Athleticism and Fitness: Woods' dedication to physical fitness and athleticism has transformed the way golfers train and prepare. He has demonstrated the value of strength, flexibility, and conditioning in improving performance and longevity on the course.

v. Resilience and Perseverance: Woods' ability to overcome adversity and recover from setbacks has served as an inspiration to those facing personal challenges.

vi. Philanthropy and Giving Back: Woods has used his platform and influence to create positive change outside of the golf course. Through his Tiger Woods Foundation, he has supported education, youth development, and community outreach initiatives, allowing underserved youth to excel academically and physically.

Tiger Woods' inspiration and influence extend far beyond his golfing achievements. He has inspired generations of athletes, broken down barriers, and made an indelible impact on the sport and society as a whole.

Tiger Woods

His legacy will continue to inspire and motivate people for many years to come.

Overall, Tiger Woods' comeback and resurgence in golf demonstrate his unrivaled talent, determination, and commitment to the game. His ability to overcome adversity and achieve greatness on the golf course will go down as one of the most iconic moments in sports history.

7.1 Return to form.

Tiger Woods

Tiger Woods' return to form in golf demonstrates his unparalleled talent, resilience, and determination. Despite numerous setbacks, such as injuries and personal challenges, Woods has proven his ability to overcome adversity and regain his competitive edge on the course. Here are some key factors influencing his return to form:

1. Physical Rehabilitation: Following several surgeries, including a spinal fusion in 2017, Woods underwent extensive physical therapy to recover from his injuries and regain his strength and mobility. His commitment to his rehabilitation program enabled him to overcome physical limitations and return to a level of fitness appropriate for competitive golf.

2. Technical Adjustments: Woods has made strategic changes to his golf swing and technique to accommodate changes in his physical condition as well as address any lingering issues from previous injuries. Working with his coaching and training staff, he has refined his mechanics and optimized his swing to maximize performance while reducing the risk of re-injury.

3. Mental Resilience: Woods' mental toughness and competitive spirit have been critical to his return to form. He has maintained a positive attitude and unwavering faith in his abilities, even during times of doubt and uncertainty. His ability to maintain focus and composure under pressure has allowed him to perform at his peak when it counts most.

4. Strategic Scheduling: Woods has taken a more strategic approach to tournament scheduling, focusing on events that match his physical condition and allow him to peak for major championships. By carefully managing his tournament schedule and workload, he has been able to maximize his performance while avoiding overwork.

5. Improved Health and Fitness: Woods' dedication to fitness and overall well-being has been instrumental in his return to form. He has prioritized a healthy lifestyle, including proper nutrition, hydration, and recovery practices, to improve his physical and mental performance on the course.

6. Rekindled Passion: Throughout his career, Woods' love of golf has been undeniable. His return to form has

been fueled by his passion for the sport and desire to compete at the highest level again. His performance on the course demonstrates his renewed enthusiasm and dedication to his craft.

Overall, Tiger Woods' return to form demonstrates his resilience, determination, and unwavering dedication to excellence. His ability to overcome adversity and rediscover his winning ways cemented his place as one of the greatest golfers of all time.

CHAPTER EIGHT: MAJOR VICTORIES AFTER ADVERSITY

Tiger Woods' major victories after adversity are among the most inspiring moments in golf history, demonstrating his incredible resilience and determination. Despite significant setbacks such as injuries, personal struggles, and a drop in performance, Woods has overcome adversity to win major championships. Here are some notable examples of Woods' major victories after facing adversity.

1. 2008 U.S. Open: At Torrey Pines, Woods won one of the most iconic victories of his career. Despite suffering a fractured tibia and knee ligament damage, Woods battled through 91 grueling holes, including an 18-hole playoff, to win his third U.S. Open and 14th major championship overall.

2. 2019 Masters Tournament: Following multiple back surgeries and a lengthy period of injury-induced absence from competitive golf, Woods made an impressive comeback at the 2019 Masters Tournament. Woods delivered a vintage performance, carding a final-round 70 to win his fifth green jacket and 15th major championship, marking one of the most emotional victories of his career.

3. 2005 Masters Tournament: Following revelations about his extramarital affairs, Woods experienced personal turmoil and public scrutiny. Despite the distractions and challenges of the course, Woods delivered a dominant performance at the 2005 Masters, winning his fourth green jacket with a dramatic playoff victory over Chris DiMarco, demonstrating his ability to block out external distractions and focus on his game when it was most important.

4. 2000 U.S. Open: Woods' victory at Pebble Beach in 2000 is widely regarded as one of the most dominant performances in major championship history. Despite receiving criticism and doubts about his ability to replicate his success following a swing overhaul, Woods delivered a record-breaking performance, finishing 15 strokes ahead of the field and securing his third major championship of the year

5. 2019 Zozo Championship: After multiple knee surgeries and a string of setbacks, Woods regained form at the 2019 Zozo Championship in Japan. He won his 82nd PGA Tour event, tying Sam Snead's record for most career wins, and demonstrated his ability to overcome adversity and compete at the highest level well into his 40s.

These victories demonstrate Woods' ability to overcome adversity, persevere through challenges, and deliver under pressure on golf's most important stages. They demonstrate his unparalleled talent, mental toughness, and unwavering determination to succeed despite all odds.

Tiger Woods

8.1 impact

Tiger Woods' influence on the world of golf and sports in general is undeniable, transcending the boundaries of his sport and leaving an indelible imprint on society. Here are some key elements of his impact:

1. Golf's Popularity and Growth: Woods' electrifying style of play and charismatic personality have sparked unprecedented interest and excitement in the game. He has attracted new fans to the sport and inspired countless people to pick up a golf club and start playing. His influence has helped to drive golf's global growth and

popularity, particularly among younger audiences and diverse demographics.

2. Diversity and Inclusion: Woods' success as a biracial golfer has challenged stereotypes and broken down barriers in a traditionally white-dominated sport. He has been a trailblazer for diversity and inclusion in golf, inspiring a new generation of diverse golfers to pursue their goals and break down barriers to participation. His influence has spread beyond the fairways, encouraging greater diversity and representation at all levels of the game.

3. Athleticism and Fitness: Woods' commitment to physical fitness and athleticism has transformed the way golfers train and prepare. He has raised the level of

athleticism in golf, demonstrating the significance of strength, flexibility, and conditioning in maximizing performance and longevity on the course. His impact has led to a greater emphasis on fitness and training among professionals and amateur golfers alike.

4. Global Reach and Influence: Woods' global popularity has elevated him to the ranks of the world's most recognizable and influential athletes. His impact goes beyond the golf course, with endorsements, philanthropic efforts, and cultural influence reaching audiences all over the world. He has been a global ambassador for the sport of golf, promoting the values of integrity, sportsmanship, and perseverance on a global scale.

5. Inspiration and Role Model: Woods' transformation from a young prodigy to one of the greatest athletes in

history has inspired millions of people all over the world. His remarkable talent, work ethic, and resilience in the face of adversity inspire athletes, aspiring golfers, and people from all walks of life.

Tiger Woods' impact on golf and sports goes beyond his record-breaking performances on the course. He has left a lasting legacy as a trailblazer, role model, and cultural icon, changing the face of golf and inspiring future generations.

8.2 Legacy

Tiger Woods

Tiger Woods' legacy in the world of golf is profound and multifaceted, encompassing his unparalleled on-course accomplishments, cultural impact, and contributions to the sport's evolution. Here are some important aspects of Woods' legacy:

1. Greatest Golfer of All Time: Woods' dominance and success in golf have cemented his legacy as one of the greatest athletes of all time. He is one of the most accomplished golfers of all time, having won 15 major championships and 82 PGA Tour events. His influence on the game goes beyond statistics, as he revolutionized it with his talent, athleticism, and competitive spirit.

2. Cultural Icon: Woods' impact extends beyond the course, as he has become a global cultural icon and

household name. He drew unprecedented attention and excitement to golf, attracting new audiences and inspiring generations of fans all over the world. His influence on popular culture, fashion, and media has helped him become one of the most well-known and influential figures in sports history.

3. Trailblazer for Diversity and Inclusion: Woods' success as a biracial golfer broke down barriers, paving the way for greater diversity and inclusion in the sport. He inspired a new generation of diverse golfers to pursue their dreams and helped to broaden the sport's appeal to underserved communities. His influence has led to increased representation and participation in golf, promoting diversity and inclusion at all levels of the sport.

4. Athleticism and Fitness: Woods' dedication to physical fitness and athleticism transformed the way golfers train and prepare. He raised the athleticism bar in golf, emphasizing the importance of strength, flexibility, and conditioning in maximizing performance and longevity on the course. His influence has increased the emphasis on fitness and training among both professional and amateur golfers.

5. Inspiration and Role Model: Woods' transformation from a young prodigy to one of the greatest athletes in history has inspired millions of people all over the world. His remarkable talent, work ethic, and resilience in the face of adversity inspire athletes, aspiring golfers, and people from all walks of life. He demonstrated the power of determination, perseverance, and self-belief in achieving greatness against all odds

Overall, Tiger Woods' legacy in golf is unparalleled, having left an indelible mark on both the sport and society at large. His legacy will live on for generations, inspiring future athletes and profoundly shaping the future of golf.

Chapter nine: influence on golf

Tiger Woods has had a massive and far-reaching impact on the game of golf, shaping it in a variety of ways and leaving a legacy that goes beyond his on-course accomplishments. Here are some important aspects of Woods' impact on golf:

1. Increased Popularity: Woods' introduction to the golf scene in the late 1990s coincided with a surge in the sport's popularity. His dynamic playing style, charismatic

personality, and record-breaking achievements captivated fans all over the world, attracting new audiences and driving television ratings and tournament attendance.

2. Globalization: Woods' global appeal and success contributed to the internationalization of golf, allowing it to reach new markets and audiences. He inspired a new generation of young golfers from various backgrounds to take up the sport, resulting in increased participation and interest in areas outside of traditional golfing hotspots.

3. Youth Engagement: Woods has had a significant impact on youth golf engagement, inspiring countless children and teenagers to pick up a club and pursue their passion for the game. His influence extends beyond the

professional ranks, as he has been a role model and mentor to aspiring golfers of all levels, inspiring them to work hard and dream big.

4. Technological Advancements: Woods' success and popularity were accompanied by rapid advances in golf equipment and technology. His demand for precision and performance compelled manufacturers to innovate and create cutting-edge equipment that maximized distance, accuracy, and consistency for players of all abilities.

5. Fitness and Training: Woods' emphasis on physical fitness and conditioning changed the way golfers approached their training and preparation. His emphasis on strength, flexibility, and athleticism raised the bar for golf fitness standards, motivating players to prioritize

their health and fitness to improve their performance and longevity on the course.

6. Increased Prize Money and Sponsorship: Woods' star power and marketability raised the profile of professional golf, resulting in more prize money, sponsorship opportunities, and endorsement deals for players on the PGA Tour and other tours. His influence helped to raise the financial stakes in professional golf, attracting top talent from all over the world.

Overall, Tiger Woods has had a profound and multifaceted impact on golf's culture, economy, and global appeal. His legacy will inspire future generations of golfers while also contributing to the game's ongoing growth and evolution.

9.1 cultural impact

Tiger Woods' cultural impact extends far beyond golf, influencing popular culture, society, and our perceptions of athletes and sports. Here are a few important aspects of his cultural impact:

1. Breaking Barriers: Woods broke down racial and cultural barriers in golf, challenging stereotypes and paving the way for increased diversity and inclusion in the sport. As a biracial athlete in a predominantly white sport, he became a symbol of progress and opportunity, motivating a new generation of diverse athletes to pursue their goals.

2. Global Icon: Woods' global appeal crosses borders and cultures, making him one of the world's most well-known and influential figures. His golfing success, combined with his charisma, marketability, and philanthropic efforts, has propelled him to the status of a global icon, with fans and admirers spanning continents and cultures.

3. Mainstream Media Coverage: Woods' dominance and star power drew unprecedented media attention to golf, raising its profile and presence in mainstream media outlets. His every move, both on and off the course, made headline news, resulting in increased interest and coverage of golf-related events and stories.

4. Fashion and Style: Woods' impact extends beyond golf into the worlds of fashion and style. On Sundays, his signature red shirt and black pants ensemble became iconic, representing clutch performances and victory celebrations. Woods' endorsement deals and collaborations with top apparel brands have also influenced golf fashion trends.

5. Advertising and Endorsements: Woods' marketability and appeal to advertisers have propelled him to the top ranks of celebrity endorsers worldwide. His endorsement deals with major brands and corporations have generated millions of dollars in revenue while also increasing his cultural impact as a global brand ambassador.

6. Philanthropy and Social Impact: Through his Tiger Woods Foundation, Woods has made significant contributions to education, youth development, and community outreach. His charitable efforts have helped to create opportunities for underserved youth and promote positive change in communities all over the world.

Tiger Woods

Overall, Tiger Woods' cultural impact extends beyond sports, leaving a lasting legacy that benefits society as a whole. His impact on diversity, media, fashion, advertising, and social change has left a lasting impression on the world, shaping perceptions and inspiring future generations for years to come.

Chapter ten: philanthropy

Tiger Woods' philanthropic efforts have had a significant impact in a variety of areas, including education, youth development, community outreach, and disaster relief. Here are some important aspects of Woods' philanthropy:

1. Tiger Woods Foundation: Established in 1996 by Tiger Woods and his father, Earl Woods, the Tiger Woods Foundation aims to empower underserved youth through education, college access, and youth development programs. The Tiger Woods Learning Center, the foundation's flagship program, offers educational and enrichment opportunities to students in

low-income communities, assisting them in developing the skills and confidence required for academic and personal success.

2. College Access Programs: The Tiger Woods Foundation's college access programs are designed to remove barriers to higher education and provide pathways to college and career success for underserved students. The foundation helps students from disadvantaged backgrounds achieve their academic goals and gain access to higher education opportunities through scholarship programs, mentorship initiatives, and college readiness workshops.

3. STEM Education: Woods is a strong supporter of science, technology, engineering, and mathematics

(STEM) education, emphasizing the importance of these fields in preparing students for success in the twenty-first-century workforce. The Tiger Woods Foundation's STEM programs provide students with hands-on learning opportunities, exposing them to real-world applications of STEM concepts and inspiring them to pursue careers in STEM fields.

4. Youth Improvement: notwithstanding scholastic help, the Tiger Woods Establishment focuses on all-encompassing youth advancement, giving understudies open doors for self-improvement, initiative turn of events, and character building. The foundation helps students cultivate their potential as future leaders and change-makers by providing leadership workshops, career exploration programs, and extracurricular activities. These activities help students develop essential life skills. 5. Local area Effort: Woods has been effectively engaged with different local area outreach drives and altruistic undertakings all through his

profession, supporting associations and causes that line up with his magnanimous qualities. He has demonstrated his commitment to making a positive impact beyond the golf course by donating time, resources, and money to support initiatives like disaster relief, military support programs, and youth sports organizations.

By and large, Tiger Woods' generosity mirrors his devotion to offering in return and affecting the existence of others. Through his establishment and beneficent endeavors, he has enabled incalculable people and networks, leaving a tradition of effect and social change that reaches a long way past his accomplishments in golf.

10.1 business ventures

Throughout his career, Tiger Woods has pursued a variety of business ventures, utilizing his brand, influence, and expertise to pursue opportunities outside of golf. The following are significant Tiger Woods-associated businesses:

1. TGR Adventures: TGR Adventures is Tiger Woods' business undertaking, enveloping a different arrangement of speculations, organizations, and adventures across numerous ventures. TGR Adventures centers around distinguishing key open doors in regions like cordiality, land, customer items, and content creation.

2. Designing Golf Courses: Woods has ventured into the design of golf courses, collaborating with renowned developers and architects to construct world-class courses. His plan theory underlines key design, ecological maintainability, and playability, mirroring his bits of knowledge and encounters as an expert golf player.

3. Restaurant and Hospitality: Woods has partnered with hospitality companies to develop restaurant and entertainment concepts inspired by his love of food, sports, and socializing. These ventures offer patrons a unique dining and social experience, often incorporating elements of golf and sports culture into the ambiance and decor.

4. Apparel and Merchandise: Woods has collaborated with leading apparel brands to develop signature clothing lines and merchandise collections. His brand partnerships encompass golf apparel, footwear, accessories, and lifestyle products, catering to golfers and fans alike with high-quality, performance-driven offerings.

5. Endorsements and Sponsorships: Woods has secured lucrative endorsement deals and sponsorships with leading brands and corporations, spanning a wide range of industries including sports equipment, financial services, luxury goods, and technology. His endorsements and sponsorships have generated substantial revenue and exposure for both Woods and his partner brands.

6. Media and Content Production: Woods has explored opportunities in media and content production, partnering with digital platforms and production companies to create original content and programming centered around golf, sports, and lifestyle. These ventures leverage Woods' expertise and influence to engage audiences and create compelling storytelling experiences.

Overall, Tiger Woods' business ventures reflect his entrepreneurial spirit, strategic vision, and dedication to excellence outside of the golf course. Woods has built a multifaceted business empire by diversifying his interests and pursuing opportunities across industries, extending his influence and impact far beyond the fairways.

Conclusion

Finally, "Tiger Woods: The Making of a Legend" exemplifies one of history's greatest athletes' incredible journey. From his humble beginnings as a young prodigy to his unprecedented success and lasting legacy, Woods' story is one of determination, resilience, and unrivaled achievement.

Throughout the pages of this book, we've looked at Woods' extraordinary career, examining the defining moments, triumphs, and challenges that shaped his path to greatness. We've seen his meteoric rise to fame, his dominance on the golf course, and his long-lasting influence on the sport and society as a whole.

Aside from the trophies and accolades, Woods' story is one of inspiration and redemption. Despite setbacks and adversity, he has consistently demonstrated his ability to overcome challenges and defy expectations. His unwavering determination, mental toughness, and unwavering pursuit of excellence have distinguished him as a true legend in the game.

As we reflect on Woods' journey, we are reminded of the power of perseverance, the value of self-belief, and the limitless potential that each of us possesses. Whether on the golf course or in life, Woods' story is a source of hope and inspiration for aspiring athletes, dreamers, and anyone striving to achieve their goals despite adversity.

In conclusion, "Tiger Woods: The Making of a Legend" honors not only one man's incredible accomplishments but also the enduring spirit of human resilience and the lasting legacy of a true sporting icon. As we turn the final page, we are filled with admiration, respect, and gratitude for Tiger Woods' indelible impact on the world of sports and beyond.

www.ingramcontent.com/pod-product-compliance
Lightning Source LLC
Chambersburg PA
CBHW050818260726
48660CB00004B/1495